PROSTATE CANCER

My Story of SURVIVAL

Bryan Norford

to Ed.
Bryan S Norford.

The Pebble Press
Lethbridge Canada
www.pebblepress.ca

Copyright © 2012 Bryan Norford

All rights reserved. No part of this publication may be reproduced, stored in a retrieval system, or transmitted in any form or by any means—electronic, mechanical, photocopy, recording, or any other—except for brief quotations in printed reviews, without prior permission from the publisher.

All Scripture references are taken from the Holy Bible, New International Version, Copyright © 1973, 1978, 1984 by the International Bible Society. Used by permission of Zondervan Publishing House.

ISBN-13: 978-0-9879352-3-6

The Pebble Press
pebblepress.ca

*Dedicated to the surgeon and medical professionals
who assisted me through my prostate cancer journey.*

Other books by Bryan Norford:

Happy Together: Daily Insight from Families from Scripture
    (with Ann Norford)
Guess Who's Coming to Reign: Jesus Talks about His Return
Gone with the Spirit: Tracking the Holy Spirit through the Bible
Anointed Preaching: The Holy Spirit and the Pulpit
Getting to Know You 1: Seeking God in the Old Testament
Getting to Know You 2: Finding Christ in the New Testament
Jesus: Is he Really God? Does it Really Matter?

CONTENTS

	About this Book	1
1	The Warning Shot	3
2	An Uncomfortable Probe	9
3	Learning the Results	15
4	The Waiting Game	21
5	The Tests	27
6	The Treatments	33
7	The Decision	39
8	Waiting Again	45
9	A Helpful Distraction	51
10	The Pre-Op	59
11	The Operation	65
12	Recovery	71
13	Leaving Hospital	77
14	Recuperation	83
15	Moving On	89
16	Outcomes	95
	Timeline	101
	About the Author	103

ABOUT THIS BOOK

This is my story. Others may be different. Cancer comes in many forms and each is a tragedy. As the leading cancer among men, prostate cancer is widespread, as prevalent as breast cancer among women. It is a fearsome prospect for any man diagnosed with it, and many families face uncertainty about life and health from this disease alone. Various means of treatment, depending on the type and extent of the cancer, can be found on medical websites or from your own doctor, and are not appropriate for this book. This is one man's story.

While prostate cancer is generally thought of as an old man's disease, younger men are increasingly affected by it. It used to be said that men die *with* prostate cancer, not *from* it. Currently, it kills one in seven Canadian men, mostly over 65 years of age as most contract this cancer in later years. Although it is frequently a slow moving disease, it will kill younger men if not diagnosed early. It is not to be taken lightly. It afflicts 25,500 Canadian men each year and my advice to all men over forty is to take a simple test. Prostate Specific Antigens (PSAs) can be detected from a blood sample and may give advance warning of the disease. Any doctor who values prevention will provide it.

Therefore, I want to share with you my experience of the diagnosis, treatment, and recovery from prostate cancer. While it is a male disease, if a man infected is married, it affects the wife as much as, often more than, the husband who has it. If he has an extended family, many more can be involved. As this book will show, a devoted wife is a strategic asset for any man facing this disease because it affects both lives.

I recorded this journey by blogging from the time I suspected the diagnosis, through surgery, and to recovery and recuperation. This provided a wealth of written memories to draw from. So all the stories in this book portray real events and people, although I changed the names of those not immediate family or close friends. The format is one of short chapters with descriptive titles that will enable you find parts of the story that interest you quickly.

What changes did prostate cancer make to our lives? How did our children and adult grandchildren respond? How did I deal with the disease and what was the reaction of Ann, my wife? What were our mainstays through this journey? You will find answers to these questions as you read. For us, our faith played a major role, and you will find occasional references to this through the book. May you find direction and comfort from its pages.

Bryan Norford
Lethbridge, Alberta
August 2012

1

THE WARNING SHOT

"You have an acute bladder infection, and high temperature," he advised me. "We are putting you on an aggressive course of antibiotics and medication to try to bring your temperature down."

The morning of Saturday, October 8, 2008 dawned clear, the promise of a fine day. My stomach woke with warning of something less. I felt a queasiness which I thought some food would settle, and had some discomfort urinating, but in true macho fashion, ignored it as something that would pass. Any chores that were calling, procrastination could defer, so I discussed my suggestion for some satisfying food with my wife, Ann. Her response was to go out for breakfast. I agreed.

There's nothing like a full egg, bacon, hash browns, toast, and coffee to start the day. It seemed the ideal answer to my dilemma. We drove ten minutes in the morning sunshine to Paradise Canyon Golf Club, overlooking the river and the steep coulee slopes that fence it on the far side. The bright, manicured golfing greens weaved their undulating way from the clubhouse to the river, and the unfolding morning looked bright and glorious. It all fooled me into thinking the day would be the same.

Breakfast appeared, as inviting as ever, but my stomach revolted as the food reached it. The earlier discomfort was decaying into some distress.

"I really don't feel well," I complained to Ann. "I don't think I can finish this." I felt annoyed at my stomach's reaction to a good breakfast.

Ann looked surprised; I never turned down a good breakfast. "If you really don't feel like it, leave it," she replied. "Let's go home and you can rest. Perhaps you'll feel better later."

That seemed like the only alternative. But driving the short distance towards home, I felt worse. "You know, I think I should go to emergency, I feel *really* sick."

Ann looked at me with some concern. "Of course. If you feel that bad we should go."

I rerouted to the local hospital and we checked into the emergency department. By this time I was shaking uncontrollably; fever was taking hold. After preliminary checks and wrist banding, I waited. A few minutes later, I was given a bed to lie on. I was cold. They gave me no blanket. I tried covering myself with my jacket.

"We didn't give you a blanket because you have a very high temperature, and we need to get it down," a nurse explained. That didn't make my body or my reaction to her any warmer.

She sent me for a urine sample. Delivering that was anything but comfortable and I returned to my bed. The nurse packed freezer bags in my armpits while we waited for the doctor. I tried to accept her sadistic treatment as in my interest. I waited once more, assuming my urine sample was being analyzed. Eventually, the attending physician came to my bed. He looked at my chart

"You have an acute bladder infection, and high temperature," he advised me. "We are putting you on an aggressive course of antibiotics and medication to try to bring your temperature down."

He left. The nurse arrived and jabbed a drip line into a vein in the back of my hand. She left. Ann and I waited some more. The process was proving stubbornly slow, and I was still shivering. A friend, Sue, a nurse who worked at the hospital, somehow heard I was in emergency and came to see us.

She scanned my charts and looked worried. "Your temperature is dangerously high," she warned me. "They have to get that down." Clearly, I had made the right choice to come to emergency. "But you're in good hands," she continued, "If you're still here, I'll check back later."

I began to feel better. As my temperature dropped, my mood was also improving. Some guilt grew at my attitude to the nurse. I *was* in good hands even if it didn't seem like it. Even if her bedside manner needed some improvement, I really had no complaint.

Time passed. Ann wondered whether she should stay, as it seemed I would be there for a while. She decided to go home.

"I think I'd better go," she said. "Call me when you need a ride home."

After a kiss, I reluctantly watched her leave.

"I'll be fine," I called after her, sounding more confident than I felt. It's always a sinking feeling for a loved one to leave you in a hospital.

Minutes later the doctor came to check on me again.

"Your temperature is going down nicely, so you're free to go home," he advised.

"I'm still not feeling a hundred percent," I volunteered.

"It'll take a while longer for the infection to clear up," he said, "But you'll be okay. There's no reason to stay here."

I didn't *feel* okay, but accepted his advice. Ann would still be driving home. I found a phone and left a message for her to come and pick me up. I just hoped she checked the flashing messages when she arrived home. I sat in the waiting room. Should I call again when she was likely to be home? I didn't. I walked outside for a while to watch for her arrival. Still not here yet. I returned to the waiting room.

Some forty minutes had passed, and as I debated with myself whether to call home again, Ann appeared from another direction with a harried look on her face.

"I've been looking everywhere for you. Where were you?" I had a flashback to similar accusations from my mother when I took too long arriving home from school.

"I've been here waiting for you." My reply was as lame as those I gave my mother.

"You weren't here when I checked a while ago," she argued.

I backtracked. "I was outside for a time watching for you to return, I must have been outside when you came to the waiting room."

She was right, and my chagrin matched my physical state. But we were glad to see each other, and left the hospital together.

"So how are you feeling?" she asked as she drove home.

"Improving," I answered, "not there yet. But I'd rather be in your hands than those mechanical types at the hospital."

"Well, they did the job, didn't they? Would you rather not have gone?"

"Of course, but I'd rather be with you," I responded, "You're much nicer to me."

"I like having you around too, and for many years yet I hope."

I wanted to be with her too. I nestled up against her shoulder as she drove. I felt at peace, her presence and warmth comforted me. I was thankful for this woman I was privileged to call my wife.

As the day continued, I felt more like my old self. "I think I should see the doctor as soon as possible," I said to Ann. "We need to find out what caused today's episode."

Ann agreed. "Call her first thing Monday morning."

Prostate Cancer: My Story of Survival

2

AN UNCOMFORTABLE PROBE

> *"Why hasn't a doctor ordered a PSA test earlier? After all, as many men get prostate cancer as women have breast cancer. I think it should be routine for any man over forty,"*

We had known our family doctor for ten years, She was younger than us, and always took our complaints seriously, giving us good advice, separating our genuine from unnecessary fears. We saw her together few days later.

I explained my bladder infection as fully as I could recall. "So, as you can imagine, we're concerned about what may have caused it." We didn't mention cancer, although we were sharply aware of the possibility.

The bladder infection made a visit to a urologist a natural response. "I'm going to arrange for you to see Dr. Hansen," she responded. "He recently located here from the Maritimes and is building up his client base, so you should be able to see him quickly."

She clearly wished to clear up any concern we had about cancer if that was not the cause. She followed up with what she considered encouraging information about him.

"He is young, just out of university for six years, so has all the latest technology at his fingertips."

While I was prepared to accept her advice—in the years as our doctor we had developed confidence in her—I wasn't sure I wanted someone close to my grandchildren's age scraping out my insides, if it came to that.

She went on. "But right now, I'm sending you for a blood test to check your PSA. Its presence in the blood is a probable sign that cancer is present in the prostate. The urologist will probably want you to have a biopsy, which is a good idea as the PSA test is not always reliable."

"Haven't I had a PSA test before?" I asked.

She checked her records. "It doesn't appear you have."

Later, as we sat in the clinic waiting for the blood test, Ann expressed surprise I had no previous PSA test.

"Why hasn't a doctor ordered a PSA test earlier? After all, as many men get prostate cancer as women have breast cancer. I think it should be routine for any man over forty," she remonstrated, "I've had mammograms to check for breast cancer for years."

"Well, you may be right about getting my PSA checked," I replied, "but 'til now I've had no symptoms whatever that might have suggested prostate cancer. And none of our previous doctors prescribed a test either. Besides, any number of things could have caused the bladder infection. It may not be cancer."

Ann still seemed uneasy. She could have suggested a PSA test herself; she was always looking for preventative measures. I could have done the same, but at that point, it was all water under the bridge. We agreed we needed to wait for test results. I was ushered into the laboratory where an efficient nurse thrust a needle into a vein inside my elbow and drew some vials of blood.

Driving home, we discussed how this unexpected event might affect our plans for the next few months. We had booked flights, starting December the 15th, to spend Christmas with our daughter in Montreal, and then fly to England for a two month spell with a mission society in southern England. Following a return stop off in Montreal with our daughter, our return home was not until early March; it was already the middle of October. But until tests confirmed the medical outcome, we made it a matter of prayer. These plans could soon be in disarray.

True to the doctor's word, I saw Dr. Hansen within a few days. He had a beard and a shaved head, *perhaps to make him appear older,* I thought. But he proved to be a personable young man, well built from working out, easy to talk to, and I felt at ease immediately. I related the history that brought me to his office.

"How do you feel?" He responded.

"I feel fine, and I've had no symptoms, apart from this bladder infection. Up to now I've had no reason to suspect anything was wrong." He reviewed with me the symptoms that could indicate prostate cancer.

"I have the PSA results, which simply state it's high, but they are not specific." He showed annoyance. "That involves another two hundred dollar test, so they avoid spending the money. I'll send you for another test and tell them to give me some numbers. Anyway, let me examine you."

He poked a protected finger where I least liked it.

"You know," he continued, ripping off his glove, "I was going to send you home, you seem in good shape. But I've detected a bit of a lump, so I think I'll arrange a biopsy—just to be sure."

I discussed with him future plans for our visit to Montreal and England. Time was passing. This occurrence was placing plans for leaving mid December in jeopardy.

"Well, one option, if prostate cancer is confirmed, is a course of hormone treatments," he explained. "With the suggestion of a high PSA, that treatment may be suitable for you. These are normally given every three months and slow down the production of testosterone, prostate cancer's favourite food."

I wondered what that might do to our intimacy; entering our seventies had not dampened our enthusiasm for that particular marriage function. I said nothing. *Whatever we might lose with that treatment,* I thought, *would be an unavoidable sacrifice if treatment became necessary.* But Ann needed to think that through as well, although I was sure of her support.

He continued; "If that turns out to be the case, I'll give you a shot before you go and when you return three months later." It seemed like a workable solution, and I appreciated his consideration of our projected travels.

The biopsy was scheduled for the 13th of November, about a month before our planned flights, further squeezing the time and uncertainty of our departure. It was

An Uncomfortable Probe

one of those medical "procedures" most of us have to endure at some time in our lives.

I checked into the hospital at the appointed time. Eventually, a nurse showed me to a curtained cubicle.

"You need to undress completely," the nurse said in a well rehearsed tone. "But you can leave your socks on."

Thanks, I thought, *that makes me feel so much better*. Then, donning the gown provided, I wondered how to tie the gown at the back. I struggled, but felt my rear vulnerable, and for which the socks were little help. Then I noticed a dressing gown was included—front opening. I slipped it on.

"Are you ready?" the voice outside the curtain asked.

"Just."

"OK, come with me."

I followed the nurse to another cubicle with an ultrasound machine and a short bed. I sat on the bed.

"Your PSA is 72.5," she volunteered, peering at the sheet in her hand. "Is that right?"

I had no idea and told her so. I didn't know whether normal was one or a hundred. Clearly, Dr. Hansen had obtained a specific number.

"Well, the doctor will be with you shortly." She pulled the curtain across and left me to my imagination which broadened as I saw the instruments lying on the desk.

The doctor was pleasant enough, speaking to me on a need to know basis. He slapped a couple of long probes together with a trigger and handle, and placed what looked like a condom over the whole assembly.

"I'm going to take five or six samples, each one by shooting a probe into your prostate. I'll warn you before each shot," he offered, presumably to calm any mounting anxiety. "Lay facing the wall with your knees up."

I took some deep breaths. I tried not to stiffen up as I felt the probe go in. Surprisingly, once the probe was in, it didn't feel that unpleasant. I wondered about my sexual orientation.

"I'm taking the first sample; you'll feel a jolt." I heard the shot, felt the impact and jerked automatically—some discomfort, but not painful. Some manoeuvring and five more jabs like that and he was done. Six small jars were lined up on his cart with their telltale tissue.

"I'm finished. You can change back to your clothes in your cubicle," and he ushered me into it. "You will have some bleeding for a couple of days, but that is natural and will soon clear up," he added reassuringly.

I dressed and drove home. I wouldn't stand in line for a biopsy, but it wasn't as bad as I had expected.

3

LEARNING THE RESULTS

"Your biopsy test is positive for prostate cancer," he began. That wasn't unexpected. "Your PSA level is high enough that, in my experience, the cancer may have spread outside the prostate."

About a week later, Dr. Hansen's secretary called to say the biopsy results were in and set an appointment for me on November 25th. Still feeling no ill effects that would suggest any sickness, my main concern was the time passing before our anticipated trip to Montreal and England. November 25th was only twenty days to our scheduled departure.

Ann accompanied me to the appointment with Dr. Hansen. He greeted us both warmly.

"Your biopsy test is positive for prostate cancer," he began. That wasn't unexpected. "Your PSA level is high enough that, in my experience, the cancer may have spread outside the prostate."

I was still unaware of the meaning of differing levels of prostate cancer. Ann wept a little. I think she assessed the situation better that I did.

He went on: "If so, the cancer will be found in the lymph glands at the base of the abdomen or in the bones or both. If this is confirmed, I recommend the hormone treatment I explained to you earlier; recall it suppresses testosterone in the body, prostate cancer's favourite food—and, most important, it slows the spread of the disease. In the meantime, I recommend a bone scan and cat scan to determine if it has spread, and if so, how far."

While I continued to wonder what effect dampening my testosterone would have on our sex life, Ann was clearly thinking of implications beyond that. But at this stage, it was unwise to be too concerned until we had more information on the progress of the cancer. We both knew whatever the outcome, we were in God's hands. We would walk through this together with Him a day at a time. After all, life would continue much as before; all that had changed is how we should handle it. Although I had originally felt it was all a false alarm, I was now prepared for either answer. Unlike Ann, I had no emotional reaction, more concerned with treatment and our immediate plans.

"As you know, we still have flights booked for December the 15th," I responded. "Should we consider cancelling or postponing them?"

"Not yet," he suggested, "I'll get you into the hospital for the scans as soon as possible and once I have the results we can make a decision." That sounded good, even if still uncertain. "If the tests show what I believe, then we can start treatment immediately. As it involves a shot every three months, we'll start the first one before you go. In the meantime, I want another PSA to confirm your previous test."

Dr. Hansen evidently wanted to accommodate our travel plans. He called the hospital later that day to secure early dates for the scans. He clearly had some pull. Then he could give the first injection, if necessary, before we left.

Arriving home, we informed family and friends—thank heaven for email! We sent a collective letter to our many friends, and individual letters to our family—three daughters and husbands, six adult grandchildren, two married. By day's end, we had many messages returned with sympathy and support—most committed to pray for us.

Our daughter Karen, who lived locally, visited us that afternoon bearing gifts—cottage cheese, pomegranate juice and flax oil to name a few—a tangy reminder that my diet needed to change. She suggested our immune system can be reinforced to respond to cancer if four things happen. First, we need to ensure a fully nutritious diet—no more wandering the aisles of the supermarket, stick to the outer circumference. Apparently the whole foods are generally found there, the junk and processed foods are found in the aisles. Second, ensure a clean local environment. Fortunately, neither of us smoke and Ann ensures the dirt I can't see no one else will see either. Next, it is important to maintain a positive attitude to fight these audacious intruders, not resign ourselves to their advance. Last, get plenty of exercise; for me usually a distraction from vegging in front of my computer. Both

Ann and Karen were solidly behind my transformation to this new regime and secretly, I was glad of it.

Our good friend Sue, the nurse we met earlier at the local hospital, joined us that evening, offering any advice we needed. She offered to contact specialists that she worked with over the years to answer any questions we had. She prayed fervently for us before leaving. With support from people like Karen and Sue the future looked brighter.

That evening, our granddaughter Jenny called. She had lost her other grandfather to stomach cancer a few years before and felt it keenly.

Not normally given to expressing much emotion, she sounded concerned. "Gramps, I'm sorry to hear about your cancer," she began. "How are you feeling?"

"Actually, I'm feeling fine. I have no symptoms, and certainly don't feel sick."

"What treatment will you need?"

"We're not sure yet. It depends on the severity of the disease. I'm waiting for scans to show the progress of the disease, which will determine the best treatment."

Jenny didn't sound convinced, "Thanks gramps. Please keep in touch, and let us know how things are going."

"Of course." After some further conversation, we rang off.

My next day started at two o'clock in the morning. It is natural for one's mind to revolve around the events of the previous day, but that was not the only reason to lay awake. My days often started very early, the time my best thinking occurred while developing a project. This book was already becoming a possibility in my mind, and I was more excited in those wee hours about keeping a journal of my cancer experience than worried about the previous day's news. Not given to much outward personal expression, the book would be an opportunity to express my own feelings and responses to the options I faced, and share my journey with others affected by the disease.

Later that morning I received an appointment for scans the following Tuesday, a wait time usually measured in months, not days. I also read my daughter Alex's blog that morning, which helped me recognize how others were taking the news. Writing about me, she said:

He waits for each moment to come, not running ahead to the "what ifs." "So, we'll see what the results say and address it then." That was his typical response. Now, more of the same. "Not the best results, but one that has good options once the next step is taken." That would be my dad. Yup . . . that would be a tear on the end of my nose.

But the most important and encouraging news came in a phone call that evening. Ann called me to the phone after answering it. "It's Dr. Hansen and he wants to speak to you."

I picked up the phone and heard him say: "I have the results of your latest PSA test, and it is down considerably to 11. You don't know what extraordinarily good news this is for you."

I recalled the 72.5 from the biopsy nurse. "Perhaps the original number was skewed because of my bladder infection."

"Could be," he responded, "but whatever the reason, this is really good news. The number suggests that the cancer may not have spread beyond the prostate. In that case, even if you were my grandfather I would suggest surgery as the best course, and you wouldn't get better treatment." To think of me as family certainly encouraged confidence in his concern for me—even if it emphasized his youth and my age.

"I have tests booked for next Tuesday," I informed him, "I assume they should confirm whether the cancer is contained within the prostate."

"Good, I will see you again next Thursday after results from the scans are available and then outline our options. See you then."

With that, he rang off.

4

THE WAITING GAME

I sense this turn in the road will have a profitable impact. As the old saying goes: "It's an ill wind that blows nobody any good." We gladly anticipate the benefits to be found in this new future together.

Apart from the original news, the next few days were encouraging. It began with Dr. Hansen's news. I still felt fine, no symptoms of any sort, and thought that must count for something. Some encounters that week were interesting, including the call from Dr. Hansen. His words: "if you were my grandfather I would suggest . . . but, of course, you're not my grandfather," encouraged my confidence in his concern for me.

A second encounter was even more interesting. I always thought bankers were pretty unemotional types. A friendly, well-informed and sensible younger lady was our advisor at the Royal Bank, and we had an appointment booked with her next day. Shooting the breeze was part of our routine, and in passing we told her of my prostate cancer and uncertain treatment.

"My father has prostate cancer, but he's not doing at all well," she informed us. "I visit him whenever I can, but he lives down east." So she identified with our dilemma.

As we were leaving, she said, "look after yourself," and gave me an impulsive hug! Then, almost as a second thought, she hugged Ann. I guess she felt an air of propriety was in order.

The appointment for the cat scan was the following Tuesday morning, December 2nd, and the bone scan was to follow in the afternoon; only thirteen days before our projected journey to Montreal and England. However, it meant Dr. Hansen would have both results at our appointment the following Thursday afternoon. This, in turn, should produce some specific steps to skewer the unwanted residents in my body, and the chance for us to leave on the scheduled date. Nothing like uncertainty until the last minute to keep life interesting.

We are blessed with a great family that cares for us and upholds us in prayer. That weekend, some of our grandchildren came just to be with us. Canadian distances reduce the opportunities for get-togethers, and we appreciated the special effort to visit with us and express their concern before we departed for England. That Friday evening, I recorded in my journal:

> Today has been a busy one, preparing for our family visit and our home group meeting tonight. It has also been run-of-the-mill; Ann at university while I continue writing to meet some self-imposed deadlines. I really don't think much about

my condition because I'm busy. Time enough for that when the scan results are in and the doctor has outlined what options we may have. In the meantime life goes on and some setback is no excuse to abandon it.

It's through times of uncertainty that our faith is tested. Are we going to run to God for comfort and shelter, or away from him because we consider he has deserted us at a critical time? This latter idea is driven by the notion that we should be able to avoid trouble because God will preserve us from it. Of course, it doesn't take much thought to realize, both from the Bible and history, that suffering is part of life. The most encouraging part of this journey is that whatever our perception, God remains faithful, he will not deny his true character.

All my life I've been seeking a nice comfortable rut to live in. Where is that simple, daily routine that doesn't change and everything is predictable? I suppose some have found it, but for us life has been an ever-changing panorama that draws energy and excitement for the challenges ahead. While we may sometimes seek a restful break, the continual newness of life keeps the anticipation alive. I sense this turn in the road will have a similar impact. As the old saying goes: "It's an ill wind that blows nobody any good." We gladly anticipate the benefits to be found in *this* new future together.

This was a time of waiting, often the hardest part of any journey. But the waiting game is God's way to help us trust. I recall the story of the lady who told her pastor she needed patience. Her pastor began praying for all sorts of calamities to befall her until she told him to stop. "Tribulation worketh patience" he responded, quoting the King James Version of the Bible that she knew so well. If we are to attain that peaceable spirit that most of us long for, being able to wait is often part of the price.

Besides, so much of the mundane in life provides opportunity for waiting. That gives us time to think. Driving, walking, household chores, and waiting rooms are time given to us to consider the important things in life, exposing our real priorities.

As planned, our grandchildren joined us for the weekend, coming because they felt the need to be with us during this uncertain time. Dan, his wife Joelle, their one year old, and Dan's brother Lee, arrived Friday evening.

"So, how are you feeling, granddad?" Dan inquired as they removed their coats.

"I'm feeling just fine," I replied. "Quite truthfully, I have no noticeable effects from the cancer. I just have to trust the tests that tell me there is something obnoxious lurking where it shouldn't."

Joelle fussed with Norah, her little one, removing her winter attire. "So, have they suggested a course of action?"

I hung their coats up. "I'm waiting for tests to find out, scheduled for this coming week." It was the best answer I had.

Joelle turned to Ann as they carried baby paraphernalia to the guest room. "It must be a worrying time for both of you."

Ann bent over, pulling back the covers on the bed. "It was a shock, but we're getting used to the idea. And we are comforted knowing we can trust God for strength whatever the outcome." She stood and turned to the others depositing belongings in the guest room. "Come upstairs when you are settled. There's a snack for you all after your journey."

The next day, Saturday, our daughter Karen, her husband Al, his mother and their adult son, joined us for supper.

"I've brought some pictures of Dan and Jo's wedding from five years ago. Are we interested in seeing them?" Al offered.

"It's been a while since we did that," replied Joelle, "it would be great to see them again."

"Most of us haven't seen them since the wedding. Let's go for it," confirmed Karen.

Al set up his computer and projector and found a blank space on the living room wall. As we watched, I pondered *our* wedding day some fifty-three years before. That had started the cycle of life that brought about this delightful event and our first great-grandchild now blissfully asleep in her crib. The hum of warm conversation around us brought reassurance of the concern our family had for us. It gave joy and hope to our hearts, and we were overwhelmed by this evidence of God's goodness. If we have to wait, what better way to do so?

But, it also made us aware of broken families or rebellious children who miss this joy, and experience the heartache of fractured relationships. Pain comes in all sorts of dress, and broken families and broken health are both part of the landscape of life. But I found it harder to be despondent about my difficulties when receiving so much bounty elsewhere. The two are just not comparable.

Dan, Joelle, and their family left Sunday morning, leaving a touch of sadness in my heart. The house was too quiet and empty when they had gone. But recalling the paraphernalia they had brought to ensure a secure and happy baby, we appreciated the effort they made to be with us. So the day was one of cleaning up, recovery, and some quiet time of required reading for the cancer war. This coming week would be eventful.

5:

THE TESTS

I'm grateful for the much maligned Canadian health system, and my experience with the scans that day confirmed my opinion. The efficiency of the process and friendliness of the staff made it almost a pleasant experience to visit the hospital.

On Monday, I awoke to read a devotional Bible verse for the day: *Man's days are determined; you have decreed the number of his months and have set limits he cannot exceed. Job 14:5.*

I really didn't need any prompting that my days were numbered. I thought about my limited time on earth the older I became; now brought into sharper focus by sickness. I had already passed my allotted three score and ten years, and now I was borrowing from someone who didn't make that number. I doubt this quote meant that my personal days were determined without any action on my part—lifestyle can have a part in the time of death—but all human life, however healthy, has limited time on earth.

For me, death is simply another deadline to meet, with certain things that I want or need to do before then. It reminds me of my previous change of life from architect to pastor. A deadline for architectural work could often be extended, but as a pastor, Sunday came whether I was ready or not! Time management was essential for that and for life as a whole. Whether my life is going to produce something worthwhile is still in my hands for the time I have left.

So what about the future bothered me the most that Monday? My disease or tomorrow's scans and their outcome? Watching television news that day answered the question. The opposition in Parliament had ganged up on Stephen Harper's minority government and forged a coalition with a majority to bring down the government. This farce played out in Ottawa: a bunch of hooligans scuffling for power, upsetting the business of the country on the pretext of putting it right, and, with dead seriousness, plunging us all into disarray. What made matters worse, 2008 was the beginning of the worldwide recession that caused so much havoc around the world. This was a time for pulling together, not for power politics. At the time, these events bothered me more than my own condition.

I was struck by three crises happening simultaneously: the world financial crisis, the constitutional crisis in Ottawa, and now my health challenge. As if in sympathy, was my body also going through a constitutional crisis because of the meagre nutrients I fed it? Hence the cottage cheese and flaxseed oil. But disease is not a simple cause and effect or we would all be held responsible for our illnesses. One way or another, my life will continue for a time yet, and I planned for it to be meaningful for the time left and for eternity. We are to anticipate both joyfully.

Tuesday arrived as it always does. I'm grateful for the much maligned Canadian health system, and my experience with the scans that day confirmed my opinion. The efficiency of the process and friendliness of the staff made it almost a pleasant experience to visit the hospital.

I arrived at nine and was sent to the imaging department, where a nurse looked at my sheet.

"Come with me," she ordered amiably, taking me to a cubicle. "Please undress, but you can leave your underclothes on." This was an improvement over the last visit, but I would still have to fight with the rear tied gown and don the dressing gown.

"When you are undressed, take a chair in the corridor here." She pointed to a line of chairs adjacent to the changing cubicle. "I will bring you a drink to dye parts of the body before your scan."

"Can I leave my socks on?" I asked. I was sure the floor was cold.

"No, but you can wear these hospital slippers instead." She handed me standard issue tie-ons.

I fulfilled all the instructions and joined a few others on the corridor chairs. We looked like a bunch of convicts in prison garb waiting to have our heads shaved.

The nurse arrived with two huge paper cups. "Drink all of this as soon as you can. We have to wait for the dye to pass through your body, so the sooner you can drink it the better."

"This" turned out to be a large cup and a half of pink liquid with the consistency of a weak milk shake. It was obviously flavoured with mint to make it half palatable, but its sluggish passage down my digestive tract made downing it a slow process. I placed the empty cups on the floor beside the chair.

She came back with another cup.

"This one is to blow your belly up to give a clearer image," she explained. "Drink it all before you get your scan"

This one was more like Sprite, went down easier and made me feel full. Shortly after, the scanner operator come from an adjacent room and called my name. I followed her into the scanning room.

"Have you ever had a scan in one of these before?" she asked.

"No." I looked at the gigantic donut contraption, with a stretcher on a track that passed through the hole.

"There's no reason to be afraid. Nothing touches you and you'll feel no pain." I hadn't imagined there was anything to fear, but now I began to wonder.

"I'm going to give you an injection to relax your muscles." She poked it in my arm and continued. "Please lie on the bed and place your hands above your head. Lie quite still until I tell you to move." I lay still but the stretcher moved, and I rode feet first through the donut hole and back.

"There. You can relax now and climb off the bed. Do you feel okay?" I saw no reason why I shouldn't be okay, but realized some who had claustrophobic tendencies might not.

"Yeah. I feel fine, thanks. I assume I'm all done?"

She looked at my sheet. "No, not quite. I see you are booked for a bone scan this afternoon."

"Yes. That's right."

"Well, you have to have a dye injection for it at least two hours before the scan. I'll have someone take you there, and then you can go home while it circulates and come back this afternoon. In the meantime, you can get dressed and someone will come for you."

"Thanks," I mumbled, and she opened the door for me.

Once I had dressed, an orderly led me to the waiting area for the bone scanner. Shortly, a nurse called me in and repeated the reasons for the injection.

"This die will make the images we take readable, but it takes two hours to reach the brain area. Once I've given you the injection you can leave the hospital if you wish until the time for your appointment."

She jabbed me with her needle. "Are you okay?" she asked after the injection.

"Yes. I'm fine," I responded. I wondered if all this dye in my body would colour me like a chameleon, or I would glow in the dark. "Am I finished now?"

"Yes. But don't forget to come back at two."

"I won't. Thanks." And I returned to my car.

Time enough for lunch. Just as well, as I wasn't allowed breakfast before my cat scan. And Ann was due at university at two. The day was panning out quite well. I dropped Ann at university and arrived at the scanning department on time. Again, I was required to change into hospital garb and a nurse called me into the scanning room.

This scanner was quite different. I lay down on a stationary bed, with a grey box immediately over my head.

The operator explained. "The box you see immediately above you contains the scanning cameras. I'm going to lower it to above your nose. Tell me if it's getting too close for comfort."

I could understand a claustrophobe becoming scared. But I assumed as long as it didn't touch or squash my nose, I had nothing to fear.

"Are you still okay?" she asked. I nodded. "If you are I'll lower it some more."

It came to within an inch of my nose—very up close and personal. Even though not claustrophobic, I felt my personal space definitely violated.

"I'm fine," I replied, *physically at least*, I thought.

"Ok. I'll start the scanner. It'll revolve around your head, but will take about half an hour. You can just relax while it does its work."

The quiet hum of the machine acted like a lullaby, and I dozed off for a while. A voice interrupted a couple of times: "Are you doing okay?" which elicited a murmured "hmm-hmm." It was a comfortable and restful end to the day's scans. Time enough to dress again and pick Ann up from the university before supper.

6

THE TREATMENTS

During the next few days we prayed about our decision and sought guidance from those who had insight to the issues.

As might be expected, the following day, Wednesday, was quieter, but not without its anticipation of Thursday's results. I woke in the night wondering about the possibilities ahead. Perhaps it's not wise to know too much as the various scenarios can lead to unnecessary anxiety. Of greater concern that day, my doctor's office was unavailable because of telephone company "network difficulties." I was not able to confirm my appointment for the next day—a little more uncertainty to test the quietness.

There's nothing like a setback to lead us into some introspection. Frequently, we will wonder if we have brought about our disease, or some other adversity. Is God angry with me? Is this punishment for something I've done, or not done? That introspection is not all bad. Our failures remind us of our innate waywardness. The more we recognize our need for forgiveness, the greater is our love for the only One who can ultimately forgive us. Acceptance of our need and his provision offers the most meaningful relationship earth and heaven afford, making the cause of our calamity irrelevant. It is on the certainty of that relationship that we had confidence in God's overarching care and direction for my adversity and those affected by it.

Ann finished her classes at the university, and began preparing for her exams. That term saw her gain most marks in the high nineties, a great boost for her ability to finish her degree—with distinction. Now she would be checking my writing instead of vice versa. We continued to pray that the appointment the next day would provide us with resolution to the uncertain future hanging over us.

Thursday, now only eleven days before our departure, proved to be as eventful as any day since the discovery of my cancer. My emotions regarding my health paralleled the upheaval over our Canadian constitutional crisis. I was still having trouble getting through to the urologist's office to confirm my appointment. It turned out I had misspelled his name and so had the wrong number. Redialling, I eventually connected with Dr. Hansens' office and reached Kathy, his secretary.

"There is no appointment scheduled for you today," she responded to my enquiry. "Dr. Hansen is in surgery all morning and booked all afternoon."

"Really? Well, have you had the reports of my scans from Tuesday?" I followed up.

"No, I've not received those yet either," she replied. "But I will check with the doctor when he returns to the office at 1.00 p.m."

I had no choice but to wait—again.

At the same time, I was watching the doors of Rideau Hall on TV. Stephen Harper, the Prime Minister, had asked the Governor General to prorogue parliament as a means of forestalling the coalition's attempt to take power. A battery of reporters awaited the future of Canada with the same uncertainty which pervaded my situation.

About 10 a.m. the phone rang.

"Bryan?"

"Yes."

"This is Kathy from Dr. Hansen's office. I've had a cancellation for 2.30 p.m. Can you make it here then?"

"Ann will be in an exam at that time." I really wanted her to be with me for that interview. But I had to take advantage of this opportunity. "But I am free to come."

"You'll be here then?" Kathy sought confirmation.

"Yes, certainly."

"Good. I phoned the hospital and they have sent me over your scan results," she added," so we're all set. See you then."

I cradled the telephone with relief. Shortly afterwards, the Prime Minister came out of Rideau Hall to announce the Governor General had agreed to prorogue parliament. The constitutional issue had been temporarily resolved—that is, kicked down the road to the next election. I hoped my issue would be resolved sooner than that; by the next day.

Dr. Hansen scanned the pages in front of him.

"Both the biopsy and your PSA level showed the cancer to be a medium risk and very slow moving. Further, the scans show the cancer to be contained within the prostate."

I greeted that news with some relief, as a worse outcome would be the cancer moving to the bones or other parts of the body.

He continued. "These are the options. I can surgically remove the prostate and this should get all the cancer. Another option is radiation. However, this has to be done in Calgary and it may be a month before you can get an interview there. The treatment could take up to several months beyond that."

Lethbridge, our home town, has since opened its own cancer clinic, but it wasn't available at that time. Dr. Hansen described a couple of other options that seemed just as unappealing.

"None of the latter procedures appeal to me due to the length of time involved, so I'm leaning towards surgery." It seemed obvious to me. "How long will the operation take?"

"About two hours."

"And how long should I expect to stay in the hospital?"

Usually two or three days," he replied. "But a difficult case could have you in four days." He went on, "If you want to go that route, let me know before you leave for England. I have a two month waiting list anyway, and we'll have you set up to go when you return in March."

"That sounds workable," I responded, "but I want to talk it over with Ann. We will try to have a decision by the weekend."

The Treatments

So, like the morning at Rideau Hall, it was all over bar the shouting! We would make a decision regarding treatment by the weekend so everything would be underway on our return. Nice neat package—at least until then. Above all, it kept our trip to England intact. Now, like the Canadian government and opposition, the next stage would be strategy.

It may seem strange while anticipating some uncomfortable surgery, I felt energized at the results—so much so that I had difficulty sleeping and spent some time around 3.00 a.m. at my computer! Even the infection that started this whole affair was a blessing in disguise, warning me of the dirty little secret my body was hiding from me. I couldn't blame my body for the cancer. It, like sin, tries to remain incognito until it has a good hold.

I reflected on my emotional response to this threat. I surprised myself at the matter-of-fact way I was responding. Shouldn't I have felt some anger, fear, or at least be depressed? Or was I fooling myself, hiding this all away in some remote dungeon of my subconscious waiting for it to surface and explode? Or was my response part of the "cold fish" temperament that Ann feels I sometimes express? Perhaps it wasn't wise to delve too deeply; I was only too happy to be who I seemed to be.

During the next few days we prayed about our decision and sought guidance from those who had insight to the issues. Our friend Sue, the nurse who visited me in my initial visit to the hospital, came to see us again.

"I've had many years working with the top surgeons in Calgary," she reminded us. "That included working with Dr. Hansen's father, and since then I've worked with the surgeons here in Lethbridge, including Dr. Hansen, your urologist."

"So what's your opinion of Dr. Hansen's surgical skills?" I asked.

Sue is particularly candid, and her reply was unequivocal. "One hundred percent."

That answer gave us the confidence to make the decision necessary for the next stage in this unexpected and unwanted journey.

7

THE DECISION

We try to find an answer or at least a meaning in unexpected events. But more than a thought process, it envelops our whole being: heart, mind, and spirit. Overpowering emotions may compromise sensible attitudes and actions.

During the next few days we discussed the options before us.

"Surgery is so invasive," Ann pondered, "and the outcome of surgery can be uncertain; you know, infections, surgery errors, and so on. Do we feel we can contend with that?"

"I'm not sure I can deal with the time element in radiation," I answered. "That will last some months, perhaps a year, and we'll be gone for two months to start with—either that or we cancel our trip to ensure an earlier start to radiation. And all the time the cancer is getting worse, and I'll probably have to put up with all that nausea."

"So you are leaning towards surgery?

"It leaves our trip intact, and surgery in March will mean it's all over then, except for the recovery period."

"If that's the way you want to go, I'll support you in it. And we'll trust God for the outcome." Ann was reacting as I had come to expect through the decades of our marriage.

"In that case, that's the way we'll go," I concluded.

So by the weekend, we had chosen surgery as the best option. That was subsequently confirmed by later events. On Monday, I dropped in to see Kathy at Dr. Hansens' office. It was one week to go before we left for Montreal and England.

"Dr. Hansen asked us to advise him of our decision for treatment," I explained, "and we decided to opt for surgery. He told us he was booked for two months, and as we are away until March, he would arrange for surgery then."

"I'm glad you have come to a prompt decision," she replied, "I've one patient who cannot make up his mind. His wife complained to me, 'If he'd made the decision it would all be over by now.' I'm afraid his cancer is only getting worse while he procrastinates."

"So you can arrange this while we are away?" I asked.

"Certainly, but how can I reach you while you are in England?"

"I'll be on email while there."

"Hmmm." She pondered. "We don't have email at the office. I'll give you my home email and we can communicate from there."

That special consideration was typical of the friendly care I had received since my first contact with Dr. Hansen. We exchanged email addresses.

The Decision

"You'll hear from me once it's all arranged. Have a great visit with your family, and we'll be ready for you when you return." She smiled encouragingly, and I left the office in good spirits.

But the progress of the disease, apparently slow moving, could probably be slowed even more by a careful diet—remember the cottage cheese and flaxseed oil!—and exercise. With regard to the former, it turned out not that bad; I found I could eat it by the spoonful if necessary! But in regard to exercise, the shepherds on that first Christmas had it over us; wherever they were minding their sheep they had quite a hike into Bethlehem. No cars or bicycles, and I doubt any sheep would have played donkey. I really don't have to hike anywhere, and it's an added chore to take time for walking, particularly in the Canadian winter.

But, as usual, Ann had the answer: walk in the university. Built into the side of a coulee, it has long corridors and many flights of stairs linking various buildings—a good half-hour workout first thing in the morning. It certainly got the lungs heaving and the blood pumping. Whether I could keep this diet and exercise up while out of routine elsewhere remained to be seen.

Not only was surgery and our journey in the forefront of our minds, Christmas was only a couple of weeks away, reminding us of the unmatched gift of God's Son to the world. But it is fitting that his birth also carries a reminder of the pain of life as well. The baby was conceived out of wedlock; not a big deal these days, but carrying an enormous stigma in the Jewish culture of the day. Mary's pain of childbirth, but also the ostracism that she would have received from most people around her, reflected the pain that this baby was to bear on the cross.

The turn of events that first Christmas was certainly something to be pondered. Mary's initial reaction reflects our response when things we do not fully understand circulate in our minds. We try to find an answer or at least a meaning in unexpected events. But more than a thought process, it envelops our whole being: heart, mind, and spirit. Overpowering emotions may compromise sensible attitudes and actions. Some people fight disease while others seem resigned to it. Perhaps an energetic response to disease will boost the activity of the "pacmen" placed to gobble up foreign bodies in the human system.

Our mental well-being depends on how we react to difficulties in life. If we recognize that adversity will certainly find us at some time in life, the better prepared we will be and the less it will disrupt our lives and those around us. We realized our greatest resource for confronting the barbs of life was placing our lives in God's hands, discovering our suffering is not meaningless and we could trust him to bring us through. However long it may seem, we knew this life is temporary; our future with him is not.

The Friday before our Monday departure packed a blizzard, providing an opportunity for packing our suitcases. The previous days had been crowded; touching base with numerous people and ensuring everything was in order before we left. Going away—especially for a three month absence—is like moving. When moving, we need to work toward a fixed deadline, making sure everything is packed, ready to go. A slow panic builds up until moving day: hope the weather co-operates, get everything on the truck, don't forget the plants outside—until the moment everything is inside the new place. The place may be a mess, but we can shut the door and breathe a sigh of relief.

Flying is a bit like that, and I felt more panic than previously—probably age catching up, or a subconscious reaction knowing the creature crouching at the door: surgery when we return from England. Either way, I looked forward to being seated on the plane knowing that it would be too late to "remember" anything else.

Ann and I were thankful for this Christmas with our daughter and family in Montreal before continuing to England. We are thankful for every day, whether in sickness or in health, as we move into the latter years of our lives, and that remained true as we faced the cancer and its results before us.

Prostate Cancer: My Story of Survival

8

WAITING AGAIN

I felt most grateful to take that journey in spite of my illness and looming surgery, and for an active procrastination that placed the unpleasant mostly on the back burner.

Three months to surgery! Waiting, not knowing the surgery outcome would probably be a most difficult time to face. We all naturally want any affair like this over and done with; the uncertainty resolved one way or another. For us, we were glad that we were not left sitting at home wondering for three months. But, never-the-less, this break away from home would be a test of our perseverance under adversity, and whether the continuing cancer might hinder my abilities—that was in addition to the effect that our age, now in our early seventies, might have on our strength and stamina.

So the prospect of surgery and its unknown consequences were always in the back of our minds, its shadow reaching into all the events of those three months. Yet, reviewing that time, I found it remarkable we received so much enjoyment from friends and family, and how our strength was sufficient for the work and challenges we faced.

Ease of travel and family connections ensured we were able to spend Christmas in Montreal and the New Year in England. None of us are angels, but we can all fly and act like them, dropping in like lofty seraphs on those we care to grace with our presence. However, I doubt the average angel has his belongings x-rayed or walks through metal detectors before he can fly.

Above all, I felt most grateful to take that journey in spite of my illness and looming surgery, and for an active procrastination that placed the unpleasant mostly on the back burner—except for the occasional sudden reminder that gave me a kick in the stomach.

In Montreal, we were able to enjoy the company of our youngest daughter Alex, her husband Gino, and Luciano, their two year old Thomas the Tank Engine addict. There were other benefits to being there. On a visit to the supermarket I discovered fruit filled cottage cheese. Perhaps the beginning of a revolution, rather like fruit filled yogurt! And I discovered it is great on pancakes. It also gave me time to continue editing our first book, *Happy Together*, planned for publishing in the spring. And there were always jobs to be done around the kids' house—most parents of adult children can relate to that.

This household was not the place to seek peace and quiet. None of the family was reserved; each of them happier with a decibeled life, although sometimes pushed to less enjoyable heights by a two year old's antics. Fortunately, Ann is also the active type that age can't dent, while I found my enjoyment mostly in watching. I took it as a compliment on my health that I was rarely asked if I was doing alright; I still felt no ill effects from my disease. At times, Luciano and I played together with Thomas and his friends, making tracks all around the living room floor; at other times, we all took trips to the shops or meals with friends. If I was to have any ill effects that Christmas, it would be from eating too much of the wrong stuff, not my illness. I was glad for health to enjoy the family festivities.

Once Christmas had passed, we packed again and prepared for our time in England. If 2008 had provided new challenges, 2009 would begin the same way. A brand new year, a brand new start—that's the general idea. But resolutions made will be broken once more, and much of the baggage from the previous year will carry over to the next; particularly personal issues: family conflict, poor health, financial strain, or private loss. Simply changing the year on the calendar would not solve those dilemmas. We would continue to face concerns from the previous year, and probably new challenges in 2009.

The purpose of our visit to England was for a two-month mission assignment with a mission society dedicated to Muslim areas of North Africa and the Middle East. We had completed a similar assignment a year earlier and we looked forward to meeting friends from the previous trip. While there, I needed to complete editing and indexing our book, and Ann had university assignments for submission. The internet enabled us to send documents back and forth to publisher and university in Canada. In addition, family planned to visit us from overseas.

Impending surgery lurking in my mind, and the intensity of our first months of 2009, would have been far more daunting without Ann's constant hard work and companionship. For a lifetime, Ann filled most of my needs for human company. I am not the gregarious type that she is, so her need for others, and my tendency to avoid them, created pointed exchanges on occasion and well expressed our happy incompatibility. But, despite our differences—perhaps because of them—Ann has been a faithful partner in all our earthly adventures for nearly sixty years of marriage. Without her, my life would have been much more difficult and a lot less exciting; my needs could have been met in other ways, but I liked it that way. I knew she would support me during this period of intensity and uncertainty, her care and love my earthly mainstay. Her unwavering closeness and exuberance buoyed up my confidence for the future; the first three months of 2009 would need it.

As we considered the challenges for the coming year, our sense of thankfulness increased, knowing many throughout the world had greater problems than we did. That thought was not a panacea for our troubles, but a continual reminder that too many faced greater adversity than ours and provoked thankfulness for the measure of health and strength we still enjoyed.

Winchelsea House on the south coast of England was an early twentieth century mansion. It had a stately grandeur that reflected the gentry of earlier years; its fading glory now converted for less aristocratic use—short term accommodation for mission personnel, local churches and retreats. Its three storeys rambled enough to disorient anyone unfamiliar with the layout. The bedrooms were huge, some with conservatories, now sheltering more beds. Larger bedrooms were divided to provide smaller ones, or reduced to make way for showers and washrooms. A huge sundeck off the top floor boasted a view of the English Channel across a small park and bowling green.

Two huge lounges recalled former opulence, space where men in their smoking jackets, swirling warming brandy in their hands, verbally put the world right without the need to do anything about it. Now, scattered couches and chairs, TV, and a stocked bookshelf, provided respite for those whose mission *was* to change the world. Three kitchens with eating areas, and a large dining room added comfort and convenience. This was the place we were to manage for two months.

In this atmosphere, perhaps I could vicariously live those days of my English youth and health again during this English break. But occasional reminders by email or kindly enquiries about my health brought my situation into sharp focus, jabbing the serenity of my musing.

Prostate Cancer: My Story of Survival

9

A HELPFUL DISTRACTION

"I must confess," I concluded, "I often think about my upcoming surgery, but I'm really surprised—and relieved—it doesn't bother me all that much. Being busy has its advantages!"

The upkeep of this residence took most of our time. After guests left, we stripped beds, laundered bedding and bathroom linen in two washers and dryers, ironed and replaced them. One washer and dryer was located in the house, the other in a laundry accessed from outside—in weather that was mostly below freezing when we arrived and steadily worsened into the worst winter for twenty years. Vacuuming took half a day, plus time cleaning kitchens and bathrooms, and supermarket trips to restock fridges. Two attached garages with supplies were also accessed from outside, while a workshop and an office with computer and printer were in separate small brick and tile buildings. Then of course, we had our own separate residence, a recently updated mews cottage (originally stables), to keep clean. Prayer for strength and wisdom was a definite resource for the work, especially on days it seemed overwhelming. The mews cottage was always a welcome retreat.

A car was available for our use; I just had to remember to drive on the right and use the gearshift on the left. Accessory levers were also reversed, and I constantly sprayed the windshield when I wanted to turn and tried cleaning the windshield with the turn signal.

Next day, half a dozen folk arrived at the house, and others followed later in the week. Because visitors came and went irregularly, some days were heavier than others. After a week was spent catching up on a month's non-use, we wondered if our plans for the coming few weeks were too ambitious. After the first week, Ann expressed concern over the workload. She took responsibility for housekeeping with my amateur help, but her hip was beginning to hurt on occasion and eventually required surgical replacement eighteen months later.

"Having a number of guests in the house is heavy enough, but you know, we are also expecting our three daughters and three grandchildren to join us here in a couple of weeks. If we have a near full house then, I'm worried we may not be able to cope. We've been busy already."

"I understand how you feel," I countered, "but don't get wound up too soon. It may not turn out as bad as we expect, the schedule gives us a few free days before then. Perhaps we can get ahead of the game."

"It's not just the workload. I'm concerned about coping with my hip as well as your health; whether we'll be able to keep up the pace."

"I feel perfectly well physically. As I've said before, my main problem, like yours, is age catching up with us, not this cancer, as upsetting as it may be. I certainly feel slower than last year, and need that afternoon nap when we can get it." I was speaking the truth, not just trying to put Ann's mind at rest. "But you let me know if your hip gets difficult. I can cover for your chores occasionally—but probably not as well as you!"

Ann recognized we were committed. "Well, you tell me if *you* have any problems, and we'll both try to get the rest we need."

"I must confess," I concluded, "I often think about my upcoming surgery, but I'm really surprised—and relieved—it doesn't bother me all that much. Being busy has its advantages!"

The excitement of the recent weeks: travel, jet lag, the nostalgia of fresh, if familiar surroundings, the anticipated planning and workload, were beginning to take their toll. We retired early that night. Streetlights through the large bedroom windows provided artificial moonlight. We lay and reminisced about earlier times, growing children, their marriages and children, during the fifty three years of marriage that brought us to that point. Uncertainty for the future added poignancy to the memories. We lay on our backs, our minds scanning the past.

"You know," Ann volunteered, "We didn't do a great job of raising our children. I wish we could do it over."

"I doubt any parent looks back without some regret," I responded. "I feel the way you do. It's a sad commentary on life."

"But I'm proud of our girls in spite of it," Ann insisted.

"I agree. We must have got it right at least fifty percent of the time. But youthful arrogance and selfishness marred so much of our child-raising—at least for me."

Ann appeared to look through the ceiling. "Perhaps," she mused, "putting up with imperfect parents prepared them for an imperfect world."

"So we can take credit for our imperfections?" I wryly offered.

"Of course not! But I believe God works through us despite our ineptitude. Nothing is lost in God's economy."

"Perhaps that is why you married me; you fell in love with my foibles."

Ann looked at me. "I love *you*," she countered, "But I'm well aware of your imperfections."

I rolled towards her. "That's what I love about you Ann. I'm so thankful to have you as my wife."

"But I'm afraid of losing you to this disease. What would I do without you?"

I realized that Ann was taking this harder than I was. For the moment, I was more troubled by her anxiety than my condition. I pulled her towards me and we embraced. The dimly tempered darkness smoothed out the wrinkles and imperfections of our bodies as we re-lived that age old instinctive ritual. Unknown to us then, that would soon be denied to us.

We had taken the assignment in England because we considered the benefits worth it; the opportunity to serve, yet at the same time to connect with dozens of family members Ann and I had in the area. Nostalgic trips to our old places of life and love, and forays into the English countryside made it all worthwhile. Not only that, our three daughters and some grandchildren were to visit us while in England, making for a great family reunion.

A week before the family were due, I woke at 2.00 a.m., and couldn't sleep after that. I slowly developed a headache around the eyes and on rising took some Tylenol. My mind was working though all the events planned for the next two weeks or so—both our family's visit and managing the guest house—starting that evening as new guests arrived.

We fear all sorts of things, and in our case, a concern that the great occasion planned with our family together here in England might go wrong somewhere. I had a fear of either of us falling; I was paranoid about things we might trip over, and my driving, particularly on the other side of the road, became more cautious. Beyond that, concerns about impending surgery for me, but also health, strength, and our age, generally made our planning more precious and urgent—this trip could be our last opportunity to visit there. Sometimes, all this comes together raising unjustified fears for the future—the immediate and the long term.

Something often happened to keep the back burner alight in relation to my prostate cancer. That Monday, an email from Dr. Hansen's secretary, Kathy, confirmed surgery at the Lethbridge Regional Hospital for March 30th, 2009. We would arrive home on the 11th, so a few days to prepare. The last day or so, Ann felt weak from the work and threw up a few times. Fortunately, I was still not feeling any ill effects from my cancer. We both felt this was probably our last trip of this type to England—we were getting too old for this game! Of course, we've said similar things before, but adventure still calls.

But those aren't the significant memories that will linger for a lifetime. We recall the generous use of a nine seat van that would take us all to visit the places of our childhood and early married life; eating together in a restaurant overlooking the beaches where we "courted"; watching our girls and grandchildren interact during and after meals (they all live great distances apart); and above all the warmth we felt in our renewed but temporary family circle. We love you all dearly.

The work was heavy but slowing down. Time to recuperate, for Ann to continue her university work and for me to respond to some publishing needs. But the events of the previous few weeks, in spite of the heavy load at times, would rank as one of the great highlights of our life.

A couple of weeks into February, I developed a heavy cold.

"Not feeling so good today, hon," I announced, lumbering stiffly down the cottage stairs.

Ann was preparing breakfast in the kitchen. "What's wrong?"

"It's a cold," I said with some resignation through stuffed nostrils. "How are we off for tissues?"

"I've got one box here. If you need more, you'd better run down to the store." Ann threw me a half empty box. "Are you sure you want breakfast?"

Her question reminded me of the breakfast I couldn't eat that had started our whole cancer journey. Perhaps she was wondering about a relapse. But there's an old saying that you should feed a cold and starve a fever.

"Sure. I'm hungry and ready for breakfast." The smell of eggs and bacon was appetizing, not nauseating. With that answer, Ann decided it was a cold and not a fever, so it was not life threatening. We sat down to breakfast together; one more of those minor fears allayed.

So for a few days, I sank into oblivion, learned to breathe through my mouth and generally milked the cold for all it was worth. I counted on Ann's skills for my comfort and support during the next few days, but her perceptiveness set some appropriate limits to any subterfuge. The cold hung on for several days. I continued to breathe through my mouth which dried out overnight and tasted like the bottom of a birdcage in the morning. I recovered. We trained the couple that came to replace us as our time in England drew to a close.

We packed, flying home via Montreal to visit our daughter and family again before arriving home in Lethbridge. It was good to be home. We spent a couple of days unpacking, opened a ton of mail, renewed expired insurances and licences, tried to remember where everything was when we left, and generally reoriented ourselves to life as we remembered it, gratefully assisted by welcome nights in our own bed.

Now, we had my surgery for prostate removal slated for March 30th and a pre-op on the 16th. Ann had some minor foot surgery scheduled for April 7th. She also had papers for an independent university study due before the end of April. Life didn't change—I was still searching for that comfortable rut. But we were thankful for the opportunities given us to serve and keep in touch with our family, in spite of the heavy schedule needed. We recognize our lives are mostly the result of decisions we have made and looking back there was little we would have done differently.

Prostate Cancer: My Story of Survival

10

THE PRE-OP

I felt like a ringed bird, and for basically the same reason. All my medical history scanned from that one piece of waterproof plastic.

If my prostate surgery was on the back burner for the time we'd been away, the pre-op placed it squarely front and centre: an electro-cardiogram to check my heart, several vials of my blood secreted away, and a battery of questions about my health from illnesses and allergies to prescribed medication—all "no"s I was glad to say.

Eventually, a nurse with a military air completed the visit.

"I'm placing this armband on your wrist, and it must stay there until surgery," she instructed.

"What about a shower—is it waterproof?" I asked.

"It'll withstand everything but fire, and if you're caught in one, you'll probably not need prostate surgery," she replied. "But come for surgery without the arm band and you'll get no blood transfusions, no nothin'."

I felt like a ringed bird, and for basically the same reason. All my medical history scanned from that one piece of waterproof plastic.

She scanned my chart for a last check. "I must say how healthy you are."

Thanks, I thought. *But not for long*. Shortly someone will be scouring out debris from my body like cleaning up a burnt saucepan, and stapling me up like a pair of old torn trousers. My dignity in tatters, I will have tubes going in to my arms and out of the most personal parts, not to mention sponge baths and being helped around like an old crock. And that isn't the end. Convalescence with some bodily functions impaired for weeks, return visits to inspect the incision and have catheter and staples removed, and the concern for possible complications. All these will probably follow surgery.

Perhaps the most amazing thing to me was that my body would eventually heal itself. after being cut up and generally messed with. The psalmist was right: God made our bodies a marvel of engineering with the ability to nurse itself back to health.

As the date for surgery approached, the pilgrimage to be undergone raised apprehensions. One day an article on Canada.com suggested that the PSA test for prostate cancer was not sufficiently reliable and many men are now impotent and incontinent because of it. Of course, it's not the PSA test itself that causes these infirmities; it's the surgery to remove the prostate that follows a positive test for cancer. In my case the PSA test was positive, but in addition a rectal exam found a lump and a biopsy confirmed cancer. However good I felt, this invader had to

The Pre-Op

be removed, but the future beyond that was not certain. The urologist claimed I will eventually retain all functions, but projections and reality do not always coincide, so I prepared for a more unsatisfactory outcome. This really was a pilgrimage.

However, my future as a whole was a lot more certain than many entering surgery for a variety of other problems, and I had little to complain about. But I could identify with the anxiety that surgery provokes in less certain cases.

Our lives continued to be busy. By then, our first book was ready for printing, and Ann was in the last stages of finishing her Political Science degree; papers to finish that month, my surgery a few days away, and Ann's foot surgery about a week later. We kept going. Nothing like being busy to keep our minds occupied.

While the busyness of the previous three months had helped to put surgery in the background, as it came closer, pictures of it flitted across my mind a dozen times a day. And the nagging questions: What level of pain will I have to cope with? How long will the after effects last? Will I be able to take care of some upcoming obligations? Add to that the necessity of buying new sleeping attire to replace the tattered shorts I usually slept in. So much to think about.

Emails began to arrive from many. I was encouraged that almost every conversation and email ended with the promise to pray for me that the surgery would go well, without complications, and recovery would be quick. I was encouraged by so many supporting us in this and other ways. We were thankful for those who provided help when we needed it; my surgery creating specific needs. It was with intense gratitude we recognized God as our final helper; the blessings of life all come from him. But we appreciated others who placed themselves in positions to act: the surgeon and the supporting medical staff that made it their life's work to help those in need.

The evening before surgery arrived with the usual regularity, even if it heralded unusual activity. I looked at my healthy body—at least healthy from how I felt and what I could see. Even discounting the disease lurking there, by next day surgery would ensure it would no longer function normally. So I had some apprehension. It was more than a trip to the dentist, and I wasn't sure how I'd feel when I woke up, or cope when released from hospital a few days later. In addition, uncertainties we cannot plan for constantly arise. I was glad my surgery was scheduled for 7.20 a.m.—little waiting time to speculate!

Ann came into the bedroom. "How are you feeling about tomorrow?"

I tried to explain in few words, but it was inadequate. "But I'm prepared. I've had long enough to think about it." I concluded.

"What about your loss of sexual ability," she asked as she undressed. "Have you thought much about that?"

"I think about it often," I replied, "but I may not lose that altogether. I'll have to wait and see. How do you feel about it?"

"I can't say it doesn't matter to me. I will certainly mourn the loss, but we've enjoyed over fifty years. I will be happy as long as you are healthy and still with me." She pulled back the covers.

I wasn't sure I could have answered that easily in her position. I slipped into bed beside her.

She rolled towards me and propped her head up on one arm. "Well, don't you want to at least take advantage of what may be your last opportunity?"

With the threat hanging over us, I wasn't in the mood. "Sorry my love, as much as I want to, I'm just going to have to pass, even if it could be the last time."

"That's okay. I understand."

With that, and even with the next day's uncertain outcome, we both settled for a good night's sleep.

Prostate Cancer: My Story of Survival

11

THE OPERATION

I lay still, feeling relieved. I was obviously alive and still functioning on a basic level. But what state was I in? I tried moving my legs, and received answering pain in the surgical area.

Up very early on Monday March 30th, we were at the hospital by 6.00 a.m.

"Have you showered?" was almost the first question an older nurse asked.

"Yes." I had showered the night before and washed what hair I still had. I wondered how many smelly bodies they had to cope with.

She checked my wrist band, to ensure the right patient was going to have his prostate removed. She asked my name and address, comparing my answers with the information in front of her.

"I have some papers for you to sign. These give permission for the surgery."

I signed the paper in the designated places, which joined other papers in a binder that travelled with me and contained all my pertinent medical information. Every person at each stage of the journey added to my history.

"Please put these hospital clothes on, and wait on the bed. I will be with you shortly." The nurse disappeared.

I was glad to have Ann with me to close those rear ties and make me comfortable. The nurse returned with a plastic bag with my name on it. *I hope that's not for my body if things don't work out*, I thought, only half in jest.

"Put your clothes in the bag and they will travel with you to your hospital ward." Ann stuffed my clothes in the bag. "I'm going to take you up to the operating room," she added. "Ann, you can come too, until he's wheeled in for surgery."

I had a choice to walk or ride, and my pride chose to walk. *I might need a wheelchair soon*, I thought, *I'll walk while I can.*

Another nurse welcomed me into the waiting area prior to surgery. She showed me to one of about eight beds, and gave me some warm blankets. Again, she checked my identification and my binder.

Suddenly Dr. Hansen appeared at the foot of the bed. He thrust his jacket front to both sides, placing his hands on his hips.

"Hi Bryan! Ready to go?" his easy manner and engaging smile relaxed me. "You'll be glad to know I'm just back from three weeks holiday; you are my first patient." He smiled broadly. I wasn't sure if this meant he was refreshed from a break, or he'd had time to forget his skills.

"See you in surgery in a few minutes." He turned to Ann. "Ann, I'll give you a call just as soon as surgery is over."

Ann gave him a number to call. "Thanks doctor. I look forward to hearing from you."

He left to dress for surgery. Shortly afterwards, the nurse and an orderly came to wheel me into the operating room. Ann and I kissed goodbye, both confident in the surgeon's skill and God's overshadowing. In the operating room, I met Dr. Hansen and his accomplices appearing to hide behind their masks.

"Can you move onto the table?" he asked, as the bed drew alongside. I shifted by body onto the table and, with professional help and some gas, was soon asleep.

Ann went to our daughter Karen's house to wait for that phone call., Sue, our nurse friend, and Marilyn, a prayer supporter, joined Ann and Karen while they waited. They shared and chatted, and spent time in Karen's pool to relieve the tension. The time dragged. Ann looked at the clock for the umpteenth time. It was 9.45.

"I expected a call by now," Ann exclaimed. "He said it would take about two hours. I hope it's all going okay."

Eventually, a call came about an hour later. Karen passed the phone to Ann.

"Ann?" the voice asked rhetorically. "This is Dr. Hansen. I'm glad to tell you the operation went well. However, I discovered more cancer than I expected, and the surgery took much longer. But Bryan is out of surgery, and you should be able to visit him this afternoon about two."

"Thank you doctor," Ann replied, "I'll be there. Is it okay if my daughter and her husband come too?"

"Absolutely. He should be able to handle that. I will look in as well to see how he feels."

He rang off. The other three looked at Ann quizzically, but her smile told them it was good news.

Ann settled on a pool sofa with a sigh of relief. "Thank God. I expected a good result, but you never know what might transpire in the operating room."

"You're right," responded Karen, the others nodding agreement. "Let's all have some lunch, and it'll soon be time to see dad for ourselves."

As I awoke, I found myself looking at a suspended tile ceiling above my bed. My eyes continually rolled backwards and a nurse appeared in my rolling field of vision.

"Do you know where you are?" she asked.

What a stupid question. Of course I did. "Lethbridge hospital." She looked relieved. She checked my monitor and left me to my thoughts.

I lay still, also feeling relieved. I was obviously alive and still functioning on a basic level. But what state was I in? I tried moving my legs, and received answering pain in the surgical area. The back of my hand had its inevitable needle and tube to a drip hanging above me. An oxygen tube exhaled up my nostrils. I checked under the bedclothes. That creation of the devil, a catheter, led outside the bedclothes one side, and another tube from my abdomen disappeared out the other.

"Where are those tubes going?" I asked when the nurse returned.

"The catheter goes into a urine bag, and the students will be measuring that every so often. We want to be sure you are urinating properly.

"What about the other tube, the one from my stomach?"

"That goes into the hemovac," she replied. I pulled a questioning face. "It's a spring loaded vacuum container that sucks fluid from your abdomen. The fluid right now is mostly urine and some blood."

I nodded. "I think that's all I need to know for now." It was as much as I wanted to hear.

"Are you comfortable?" I nodded again. "If you need anything, press the buzzer," she added, and left.

Within and hour or so, Ann appeared with our daughter Karen, husband Al and our grandson Josh. As they arrived, I noticed cards on a pin board together with a copy of the cover of our first book, *Happy Together*. That too would survive my surgery. It was a reminder that this experience was a stop along the way, not a destination.

"So how're you feeling?"

"Okay, considering what I've been through. Comfortable enough right now."

I felt sorry for them; I was ashen due to loss of blood and must have looked a step away from death.

"I probably look worse than I feel." I added.

"How's the incision?" Karen asked.

"All stapled up," I replied, "come and take a look." I pushed the bedclothes down and the dressing aside to show a row of gleaming staples doing their appointed job. Al backed away; the view not as amenable to him.

"I've brought a couple of home baked muffins for you, when you are able to eat them," Karen said as I covered up the scene of devastation. As it happened, I had no nausea and later managed some clear soup and jelly.

While the family was there, Dr. Hansen also looked in as promised.

He, in common with everyone else asked how I was doing.

"I seem to be doing alright," I answered.

"That's great," he said. "But you should know there were further lumps not detected previously and I had to take out more surrounding tissue than anticipated. This included the surrounding nerves—they may grow back in several months—and some lymph node samples to detect any possible escaping cancer cells. It was a longer than usual surgery, needing two blood transfusions during the operation. However, the surgery was successful. We'll have the tissue samples processed to tell us if the surrounding tissue was free of cancer."

"I'm just grateful it's over," I responded, "even if it was more extensive. Thanks for the surgery."

He chatted with the family for a few minutes, and went on his rounds.

Ann returned that evening, and we spent time together, both thankful that surgery was over and it appeared successful. We privately offered a prayer of thanksgiving to God, and gave thanks for the people he had placed in our lives to provide healing.

12
RECOVERY

Feeling a little more human, I worked my way back to a chair to sit for a few minutes. Not too comfortable, I laboriously made my way, with help, back onto the bed and rested. The total ordeal left me exhausted.

The morning after surgery, I was helped out of bed for a shave and wash-up. What a palaver! Getting in and out of bed proved a painful and slow business. Once standing, I had to hang onto my catheter bag, and ensure the hemovac sucking fluid from my abdomen was securely fastened to my gown.

"Bring your girlfriend with you," added the nurse, pointing to the mobile stand holding my drip feed. With all these in tow, I reached the bathroom and sat down in front of the basin.

Then I felt nauseous. "I think I'm going to faint."

"No you're not," the nurse ordered. "Take some deep breaths," and she rubbed my back.

The nausea passed and I was able to have a reasonable shave and brush my teeth. Feeling a little more human, I worked my way back to a chair to sit for a few minutes. Not too comfortable, I laboriously made my way, with help, back onto the bed and rested. The total ordeal left me exhausted. What normally took ten minutes of leisurely time, was all I could manage that day.

But the catheter—in some ways the most uncomfortable part of the whole affair—was creating soreness at the entry point. I complained about it to the student nurse. Perhaps she could relieve it.

"I'll see what we can do," she said, and brought in a couple of nurses for advice.

One nurse clearly wanted nothing to do with the area in question.

"It's all a matter of care and maintenance," she said stiffly, standing at some distance.

The second nurse was more sympathetic, and came alongside the bed. "It's all a question of comfort, isn't it? Try this cream. It should help." And she offered me a tube.

"If we give you a bowl and a facecloth, do you think you could clean the area yourself?" nurse number one suggested. She was obviously not interested in doing it.

"Yes, I think so," I responded, increasingly embarrassed by the whole episode.

The nurses left, and the student nurse came with the required bowl of warm water, placing it precariously on the bedclothes, and gave me a cloth and towel.

The old saying that "the patient took a turn for the nurse," is as idiotic as it is banal. Sickness has a way of negating any sex drive; In my case, all I had left was complete humiliation. My only interest was in recovery. Nurses, young and old, generally became surrogate mothers, who could help make it all better.

I cleaned the whole personal area as much as I could, finding a lot of dried blood left from the surgery. Obviously, no one else was interested in cleaning that area either.

I was grateful for John, a friend, dropping in later. He previously had an alternate surgery for prostate cancer and was more aware of my discomfort.

"I know exactly what you mean," he said. "I found Noxema was the best thing for that."

"Thanks, I'll try it," I responded, and later Ann brought me a big jar. That definitely helped.

The following day, Wednesday, I was instructed to take a shower. That was some operation. Just getting there with all the paraphernalia hanging off my body and the pain of movement were the first obstacles. Then a tug at my nose reminded me I forgot to unhook the oxygen. Once more, a student nurse ensured a successful foray to the shower.

Once in the shower, she found hooks to hang all my plumbing equipment, and then left me to attempt a shampoo and shower. Actually, I was surprised at how well I did, reaching most of my extremities. Out of the shower the student nurse helped me towel off and don that frightful hospital gown once more. Again, I had to swallow my pride in big gulps.

Later, the surgeon visited again. He enlarged on my surgery.

"You should know that your surgery was quite extensive as the tumour growth was worse than the biopsy had shown," he said.

"I guess that means a longer stay in hospital, more than the usual two or three days?" I responded.

"Yes, but you'll recover okay. It'll just take longer. I'll check in with you again."

The next day, Thursday, I had intense pain during the afternoon—perhaps from overdoing things. I had taken a full walk around the hospital wing, and spent some time in the chair. They were able to get the pain down; never thought I'd be thankful for morphine.

I had encouragement from several friends who checked in with me. My doctor had met the surgeon in the hallway, and she passed on his words to her that confirmed his message to me. He'd told her: "It was extensive surgery, but he's young and healthy and he'll recover." I could understand the healthy bit, but young—at 72? But thinking of the average age of patients he normally dealt with, I was probably young in comparison.

Later that day, an incident occurred that relieved the boredom, even if it caused some discomfort. My neighbour in the adjoining bed had a leg removed before I arrived. Apparently they did it twice; came back for another chunk after their first grab. He had a fine head of grey hair that needed cutting and his barber agreed to come to the hospital for it.

With his customer in a wheelchair, the barber decided that the best place to cut it was between the two beds in the room, despite my suggestion that the fluorescent light was just as good on the far side of the adjoining bed. When the student nurse came in to attend to my plumbing needs, squeezing between the wheelchair and my bed she tripped on my catheter tube and went sprawling. Not sure what came off worse: her knees or the jerk on my catheter. Fortunately, the catheter was well anchored, and the jerk was more discomfort than pain.

To add insult to injury, this resourceful barber made an off colour remark about that not being the way to catch a girl. He eventually apologized, but called me an "old-timer" which, although I probably looked the part, I certainly didn't appreciate. He finally made off with the twenty-dollar bill my neighbour gave him for a ten dollar cut. I suppose the other ten he considered travel expenses.

Prostate Cancer: My Story of Survival

13

LEAVING HOSPITAL

I could not wait for Ann to pick me up and whisk me home. Time dragged until about 11 a.m. when she arrived. Time still for the duty doctor to release me, and a nurse to come and explain the paraphernalia I needed to take home.

On Friday, I had another shower providing one more step to restored humanity, and Dr. Hansen visited again that day.

"If you wish, you could leave tomorrow," he declared. "What do you think?"

"The sooner the better," I replied.

"Okay. But you can stay longer if you feel you need to. It has been a slow recovery, and extra time here wouldn't be wasted."

"If you are comfortable with my leaving tomorrow, I would prefer that."

"Good enough. I'll arrange for the duty doctor to release you tomorrow, and you can go. Someone will arrange for home visits, and ensure you have all you need. I'll see you at my office in a week or so," and with a big smile, he was gone.

There is nothing like a stay in hospital to make you feel terrible even though the physical statistics are encouraging—a practical case of feelings overwhelming the facts. Times of discouragement randomly occurred while I was there. The beds were uncomfortable, the chairs hardly made for patients to sit in; and hospital gowns restricted movement and caught on everything. Add to this, frequent pokes, jabs and checks at all hours of the day and night made matters worse.

It is easy to see how anger can build up in hospital situations where pain and hopelessness converge. Although my situation was a passing one, it was easy to become impatient with short term progress. I found it difficult to improve strength in the hospital—the food didn't seem all that good, although I probably wasn't in a position to really enjoy it. Plus, opportunity for exercise and staff help to move around was limited. At that point in my recovery, I thought it would be served best at home, even though some medication and a couple of drainage tubes would accompany me. Apparently, a nurse would visit making sure recovery was progressing.

But this has to be counterbalanced by the kindness and dedication of doctors and staff toward their patients. My discomfort did not extend to the hospital staff, who were always friendly and efficient. I was pleasantly surprised at the number of student nurses that I met during the few days in hospital; it boded well for a new crop of nurses for the future. Despite the obvious need to impress their supervisors, I really felt their personal dedication and care.

Saturday, I could not wait for Ann to pick me up and whisk me home. Time dragged until about 11 a.m. when she arrived. Time still for the duty doctor to release me, and a nurse to come and explain the paraphernalia I needed to take home. I still had a catheter and a drainage bag from my abdomen. The nurse showed me the equipment I would take home with me.

She held up a plastic pouch with straps attached. "This is your day bag for your catheter. It straps around your calf and the catheter connects to it. This should let you get around during the day."

I tried putting it in place. It seemed workable.

"This is your night bag," The nurse showed me a bag similar to what the hospital had been using; a cheaper plastic version, of course. "Connect this to the catheter at night, and let it hang outside your bed."

"So these need to be changed night and morning?" I confirmed.

"Absolutely. But in addition, they need to be cleaned out after use, and the connections swabbed with an alcohol rub each time."

I could see that going to bed and getting up were going to be major enterprises.

"I'll see that it's done," Ann volunteered for me.

"Perhaps you'll volunteer to do it as well?" I added, smiling at her.

"Not so sure about that." She smiled back.

The nurse brought us back to technical details. "When you two have sorted out division of labour, I've one more item: the hemovac. That also needs cleaning morning and evening, and, of course, both receptacles need emptying as needed during the day. Any questions?"

Beyond how I would cope with this routine, I had none at the time, although I was sure questions would arise later as I tried to put her instructions into practice.

Shortly after she left, a home care supervisor came to see us.

"I will arrange for a nurse to visit you on Monday and see how you are doing. You can arrange with her any assistance you might need after that. Okay?"

I nodded compliance.

"Good," She concluded, "the duty doctor will be here shortly to release you." And she left.

The doctor arrived a few minutes later. "So you want to go home? Ready for a hamburger I'll bet." He handed me the release form for signature.

"Not sure I'm ready for a hamburger just yet, but give me time," I replied, signing the form, and returning it to him.

"Are you having any pain?" he asked.

"Moving around is mostly okay, but laughing or coughing is painful."

"Just don't get a cold, or watch any funny movies," he suggested. "Here is a prescription for pain killers, Tylenol 3s, in case you need them. Good luck." Then he was gone and we were free to leave.

Ann pushed me in a wheelchair to the exit, and left to bring the car up. I walked to the car, and we drove home.

"Glad to be going home?" Ann asked.

"Of course! I can see it's going to be heavy going for a while, but I'll find a way to cope with it. I am just happy to be home again with you."

Prostate Cancer: My Story of Survival

14

RECUPERATION

Healing is often two steps forward and one back; overdoing it one day and paying for it the next—it's not easy to strike the right balance.

The first weekend at home was eventful. Simply getting into some sort of routine was challenging. I decided to give myself an hour or so each morning to dress and again in the evening to prepare for bed. Certain movements were still painful, so the simplest manoeuvres took on the dexterity of a contortionist, trying to avoid the twists and turns that painfully reminded me of why things were that way.

Since the operation, I slept on my back. Laying on my side was too painful, and with the tubes coming out of my body, laying on my stomach was impossible, and if possible, probably too painful as well. My first night home, I slept well, if sporadically, and that gave me confidence we could manage. But the confidence was short lived.

Sunday night about 11.00 p.m., I nudged Ann.

"We have a problem."

"What?"

"I'm all wet."

"Yes. I can feel it. What's going on?"

We pulled back the bedclothes and found the hemovac had overflowed.

"Didn't you empty it?" Ann asked.

"Of course! Take a look."

The hemovac was almost empty. The problem turned out to be a blockage somewhere, causing an overflow of fluids and misery, and work for the washing machine. Nothing for it, but to dress and drive to emergency for a repair. Easily fixed, but we were not back in bed until 3.00 a.m.

As I undressed Monday evening, I called to Ann.

"Ann, we have a problem."

"Oh no! What is it this time?"

"The exit wound for the hemovac line looks infected."

"We'd better get back the hospital again," responded Ann. "We can't let that develop."

She was right. Nothing for it, but to dress and drive to emergency again. That produced a couple of vials of antibiotics and another late night. Healing is never a straight line.

However, despite the setbacks and a couple of broken nights, by Tuesday, I was feeling much more in control, able to cope with the latest life games within some sort of organized framework. That was just as well, as Ann went to Cardston for her surgery that day to have a bunion removed; friends kindly drove her there and back. I had the house more or less to myself, so it was a God-given (forced?) opportunity to make sure that I could cope reasonably with the daily round.

During the day, John, who had suggested the Noxema for my catheter soreness, looked in with this wife Joanne to see how I was doing by myself that day. Joanne was a nursing instructor. During their visit, I had a bout of coughing—quite painful—but Joanne had the answer. She picked up a nearby cushion and pressed it against my stomach.

"That should soften the pain some. Let the cushion absorb the movement," she advised. It certainly helped.

Ann arrived home about 7.00 p.m. quite elated. The cause of her elation? On arrival in the operating room, she was given a choice of general anaesthetic or an epidural (spinal injection) and she chose the latter; she was quite proud of herself. The surgeon chatted away while fixing her toe, although she found the sound of the saw disturbing.

So the following morning we were slow moving at first, but by noon Ann was walking—carefully—on the foot without even the support of a cane. I'd had a good day previously, but not feeling so good that day. That time in our lives and health conditions was not the place of laughter and joy—at least not all the time. Mind you, even in the difficult circumstances, we did see the funny side of things quite frequently, and that helped keep us sane. We had lived a busy lifestyle to that point—after all, we were still in our early seventies, but to see us that morning, it looked as though we already had one foot in the grave. Healing is often two steps forward and one back; overdoing it one day and paying for it the next—it's not easy to strike the right balance. Fortunately, we had the option of doing only necessary things, and took things easy that morning.

That afternoon, I was scheduled to have the hemovac tube and staples holding my abdomen together removed. A cause for celebration. As both Ann and I were unable to drive—the exertion too painful for me, and Ann's driving foot was still too sore—friends agreed to take me to the hospital.

I hadn't seen Dr. Hansen since the hospital stay.

"Hey, good to see you again. How're you doing?" he asked

"Managing reasonably well," I replied, "but only too happy to have this hemovac bag removed."

He looked at the bag. It was almost empty. "How long since you emptied it?"

"Early this morning."

"Well, you are obviously losing so little, I think we can get rid of it,"

I laid on the bed, and he removed the tube from my stomach.

"I think we can do without these now, as well," he said, referring to the staples, and removed them also.

I had a sense of exhilaration, being freed of some hindrances, although I still had the catheter. But the tube exit wound was bleeding a little.

"Let's see if I can find a dressing for that," Dr. Hansen said, and rummaging around the room, finally found one, stuck it in place with some adhesive tape, and I was ready to go.

Recuperation

That first week at home took us to the Easter weekend. Life was still hampered by a catheter, but I learned to cope with it until April 20th when it was removed. Meantime, ablutions and a shower plus the shenanigans necessary to survive my post surgery world took an hour or so each morning. Then I needed time to rest! Returning strength would take time, but was progressing.

It was only three days since Ann's foot surgery, but the fine weather called her into the garden where she pottered happily; that, after a morning littering the kitchen as she cooked up a storm. My appetite didn't take too long to return.

But Easter, traditionally the period remembering Christ's death and resurrection, had particular meaning for me following surgery. It feels a little peculiar to think that I had someone else's blood flowing through my arteries and veins during surgery. Although I had been a blood donor most of my life, I was particularly grateful for the one who donated blood for me. The parallel is all too clear: I am eternally grateful for the blood that was given for me at the cross. Human blood gives me existence, but the life that has ultimate meaning for me is the transcendent life gained through the blood of Jesus Christ shed for me.

We were invited out that Easter weekend for supper both days. Monday was an unexpected down day following the weekend invitations and overdoing it. That discomfort affected my thinking; I felt deeply discouraged and struggled to the deck to enjoy some early mild weather. But the discomfort had the better of me: I broke down and cried. But that didn't last long—it was too painful! In addition to the pain of much movement, all the nerves around the abdomen rattled for attention as they recovered from surgery. They insistently demanded recognition by continually itching. I found it hard to discipline myself for healing, when there was so much else I wanted to do.

But even that time aside was not without its usefulness. If nothing else, it taught patience—again! It would pass if I was prepared to wait. A nurse friend suggested healing from surgery generally takes six weeks—another four weeks of slow, if steady, healing. This was one truth I was not really interested in buying, but couldn't avoid either!

On Tuesday, Ann had her foot bandages changed. For the last few days they hadn't held her back anyway, except she wasn't able to drive. That afternoon, Ann took off with the car to run errands; she was practically back to normal. My recovery from surgery would take longer.

15

MOVING ON

Healing comes both through exercise and rest; exercise to stretch the body and rest to allow it to recover. We still had not adjusted the balance between exercise and rest. The temptation to get back to normal was too seductive.

The following weekend, three weeks from surgery, was an adventure; my first foray for any distance from home. We had registered to attend a writer's conference in Calgary, about two hundred kilometers north, and still planned to attend, even with my close abiding catheter still in place. We stayed with our granddaughter Jenny and husband, learning to cope with the inconvenience of recuperation in a home other than our own. The surgery was still uncomfortable at times, and the bag on my leg made walking any distance difficult. But I found being absorbed in the conference mitigated these discomforts.

This event marked the beginning of a new phase in our lives: writing books on subjects close to our hearts. We had a proof copy of our new book *Happy Together: Daily Insights for Families from Scripture*. The conference was an opportunity to commence promotion and gauge interest. Ann looked forward to completing her Bachelor of Arts degree in Political Science at Christmas that year, and I had a second book on the go with others lurking in the back of my mind. We were excited at the possibilities that a combination of practical theology and political theory could conjure up as we considered the problems facing people in Canada and the world.

Following that weekend, completed with some discomfort but no major setback, we were set for the final phase directly related to our surgeries. Monday, as scheduled, a young nurse came to remove my catheter. The procedure was quick and painless, if another embarrassing event.

"Now you'll find it will take some time to regain the use of your urinary muscles." She warned.

"How long might that take?" I asked.

"It'll probably take a few weeks." Her answer turned out to be woefully inadequate. "If you have any trouble in the meantime, let me know. You will, however, need some pads until you gain use of the muscles."

That didn't impress me a whole lot. I pictured myself back to babyhood, wearing diapers. But I had no alternative, and found male pads in the local pharmacy. They would fill up irregularly, requiring a extra one within reach for replacement. That didn't stop the occasional flood; easily dealt with at home, but totally embarrassing on a visit to a friend. I had to borrow a pair of her pants to return home. I had to consider this part of the healing process, despite its inconvenience.

Wednesday that week, I had my appointment with Dr. Hansen, delighted I was able to drive to his office. He entered the consulting room with his usual smile.

"How are you doing today?

"Still some discomfort moving about, but definitely improving," I replied.

"It'll take a while, especially as it was major surgery. I took out a lot of surrounding tissue when I discovered the extent of cancer in the prostate. That has all been sent to the lab for testing."

"How long will that take?"

"The amount I sent will take some time, but we should have an answer within a week or so. Your doctor will contact you with the result."

He changed the subject. "You should know that the tissue I removed contains the nerves that connect the brain to the penis. You may be sexually aroused but the penis will not get the message. Have you had difficulty getting an erection?"

"Up to now I've not really been in the mood, and I've had a catheter in until two days ago. That didn't help either."

"Well, considering the amount of tissue I removed, it's unlikely the nerves will grow back—but they may, you never know." He handed me some packages. "Try these samples, they may help."

The packages contained Viagra and similar stimulators.

"Thanks. I'll try them."

"If they don't work, we can try something else."

We set the next appointment for a month's time.

Ann had not been with me for that interview, so we had the inevitable conversation when I returned.

"So what did the doctor say? Is he pleased with your progress?" were her first questions.

"Progress is good," I reported, "and we are awaiting test results of the tissues he removed. But we also discussed sexual activity, and that was not so good."

"You're having difficulty getting an erection, aren't you?" she observed. "Is that going to be a problem?"

"It may be, and things are not looking up for me right now," I grinned self-consciously at my oblique reference. "But Dr. Hansen has given me something to try—you've heard of it: Viagra." We had never needed help before and were active up to my surgery.

"You know it doesn't matter to me if we can't express our affection that way again; there are many other ways. I'm more interested in you being with me for a long time yet." Ann was unequivocal.

As it happened, Viagra and the like, needed those missing nerves to work, so they all went in the garbage. Ann's "many other ways" would be sought and cherished.

The next day, Ann had a final trip to her surgeon and her foot was declared good to go. This meant that we were both back to a primitive version of normal, following surgery. But the following Sunday four weeks after surgery, was not a good day. We went to church in the morning, but I felt weak and had pain in the surgical area. The following day, I felt less well than a week earlier. We were obviously getting back into routine too quickly and my body complained as a result. Healing comes both through exercise and rest; exercise to stretch the body and rest to allow it to recover. We still had not adjusted the balance between exercise and rest. The temptation to get back to normal was too seductive.

The following weekend, however, was the reverse. For the first time I felt like my old self since the surgery five weeks before. Not that I was out of the surgical woods yet, and it would be a few more weeks until I regained full strength, but it felt significant and I was encouraged. I considered this evidence of God's grace and gifts. The ability of the body to heal itself is a gift of God, for he is the creator and ultimate healer. Prayer was a gift of God's grace, not only for me, the recipient of those prayers, but also for those who prayed.

Especially, I was grateful for the continuous support and encouragement from Ann; her gifts continued to be the grace of God towards me. 2010 would be our fifty-fifth year of marriage. We could both look back to God's overarching care for a lifetime.

Prostate Cancer: My Story of Survival

16

OUTCOMES

"With the original PSA over 70, without treatment, you may have had serious or significant problems from the cancer," he confided, "or might even have died from complications related to the cancer by now."

About mid April I had my next meeting with Dr. Hansen. I had met earlier with my doctor who indicated that the tests on my tissues were clear of cancer. Did this mean I was healed?

Dr. Hansen greeted me with: "You're a cancer patient now, so I'll be keeping tabs on you regularly. I'll be seeing you every three months, and if there is no recurrence, eventually once a year."

That made me think. This was not a once in a lifetime occurrence, but ongoing vigilance to ensure no relapse.

He went on, "We'll take blood samples each time to see if there's any change in your PSA. Right now it's zero."

"I understand the tissue tests were negative. Does this mean I am now clear of cancer?" I asked.

"There is no certainty with cancer," he replied, "but your chances of it coming back are less than forty percent, closer perhaps to twenty-five. That's why we will keep checking."

"OK. I understand." I changed the subject. "I tried Viagra and the other stimulants you gave me, but they had no effect."

"I suspected as much. There is a drug you can inject directly into the penis. Would you like to try that?"

That did not seem like a pleasant prospect, but perhaps worth a try. He gave me a prescription. That was as much of a dud as it was unpleasant, so that went the way of the previous efforts. Ann and I resigned ourselves to a change of life. Unexpectedly, the actual loss seemed less of a problem than the expectation of that loss prior to surgery. Was that a result of advancing age, less desire as a result of surgery, or prayer about the issue? Probably a combination of all three, but whatever it was, it eased our move into a new phase of marriage.

Now, I found just being with Ann, nestling against her on the couch or in bed, gave enormous satisfaction. We were both grateful to be together still, although the experience had reminded us that it would not always be so.

Concurrently, my ability to control urination improved. After about three months, I had control for most of the time. But physical effort still caused leaking, for which I scoured the pharmacy shelves for a more comfortable answer. Assorted pads for females—light, heavy, long, short, thick, thin, with other variations for the female form took up metres of stacked shelving. Girls were clearly not as squeamish as men about their needs. But no resources for men were available other than bulky attire, presumably to maintain liquid from whichever direction the wind blew. Clearly a case of female bias, I was not to be outdone, and sheepishly scrutinized the female shelves for a smaller pad for experiment. They displayed a rich variety the fair sex desired and, after some experiments, provided the convenience and assurance I required.

After a few months, the incision healed, and life was almost back to normal, except for the variations surgery had created. During the next year, visits to the surgeon showed the PSA continued to be undetectable. On a visit a year or so later, Dr. Hansen shared that he thought he had given me a sentence of death with the first results on our initial visit to him.

"In fact, with the original PSA over 70, without treatment, you may have had serious or significant problems from the cancer," he confided, "or might even have died from complications related to the cancer by now."

That was a fresh reminder of the fragility of life, and the need to be prepared for death. I realized anew personal affairs needed to be in order, so that either of us could continue alone. But most important, we were prepared for life after death, having had that assurance since our teen years.

Later, eighteen months after surgery, we had another reminder of life's brittle nature: I had a severe heart attack. This was one week before Ann was scheduled to have a hip replacement, which reflected our desire to do everything together. Once more, I was impressed with our Canadian health service. Within twenty four hours I was stabilized and had a stent inserted into a blocked artery to the heart.

I was home again three days before Ann went for surgery. All three daughters came to see us, one local, one from Montreal, and the other from New Zealand, a delightful time together during the next two weeks as we recovered. Our daughter Heather, a geriatric nurse, cared for us during those two crucial weeks. As she left, friends drove us to Edmonton for another writers' conference, much to our daughters' concern. I had recovered well, and Ann hobbled with a cane for a couple of months before she resumed her usual life.

I continued to have regular check-ups with the surgeon, each one preceded with a blood test to measure my PSA. Two years after surgery, Dr, Hansen noted an minor uptick.

"Your PSA shows 0.2," he announced, "nothing to be alarmed about, but something we should keep an eye on." He went on. "Surgery now is out of the question. If there is a cancer cell lurking somewhere we don't know where it is. However, the chance of any serious concern is probably ten years away."

"That would put me into my mid eighties," I responded. " I suppose if I was already eighty-five, it would be less of a concern?"

"Yes, that's right. In the meantime, if we do see any unusual activity we can look at the alternative, which is radiation. "

"What about chemotherapy?" I asked.

"Not for this cancer. Radiation is the only alternative. If you like, I can arrange for a meeting with a radiation oncologist to review the procedure."

By this time, Lethbridge had opened its own cancer clinic and an appointment was arranged. That meeting was interesting. This doctor was very formal in her presentation, quite different from Dr. Hansen's casual and empathetic approach. She was there to inform, not discuss. She insisted I was taking medication for high blood pressure. I had never had high blood pressure in my life; the medication was to ward off future heart attacks. She also echoed the rivalry between some medical professionals.

"Surgeons always want to operate," she said, intimating radiation in the first place would have been preferable.

But she provided useful basic information, filling gaps in our ignorance, a first step in allaying fears. Besides, I felt that radiation was a distant possibility if necessary at all, and who knows what alternative treatments might be available then? My next check up measured my PSA at 0.3, three years after surgery. Again, something to be watched, but of little immediate concern.

But what of the future? Making the most of the time left to us was paramount. What were our priorities? Now we had a family of twenty; consisting of our three girl's families and three great grandchildren. Having been initially responsible for bringing them into the world, we felt a corresponding desire to provide whatever guidance our experience and a lifetime of gathered knowledge would provide. Having good relationships with all the family, it was a delight to be with any of them. But was there a legacy for their lives beyond ours we could leave them?

Any legacy would not be money. We had enough to live out our retirement years and not much else. A greater legacy would be our faith that sustained us through life. Our first book began a drive that would provide spiritual guidance for a lifetime. Later books, some now in writing, would describe much of our life as a historical resource. Also, being an introvert, it was easier for me to write how I felt than to say it. So spending time with our family now became a routine; not easy, as they are scattered around the planet and we travel, not to see the world, but to be with those we love.

So three years after my prostate surgery, Ann and I share a full life of writing, encouraging young writers, family support and visits, and contact with other elderly friends; many older than us and often with debilitating conditions. It is an ongoing reminder of the debt we owe to the medical professionals that extended our life together, the gratitude we have for the family and friends that surround us, and above all thankfulness for the grace of God that has placed all these special people on our earthly pathway. We look to the future with confidence and joy.

TIMELINE

2008

October	8	Acute Bladder Infection
	14	Initial Visit to Doctor
	30	First Visit to Urologist
November	13	Biopsy
	25	Biopsy Results
December	2	Cat and Bone Scans
	8	Decision for Surgery
	15	Flight to Montreal
	29	Flight to England

2009

March	7	Flight from England to Montreal
	11	Flight from Montreal to Lethbridge
	16	Pre-op
	30	Operation
April	4	Home from Hospital
	7	Ann's Foot Surgery
	8	Removal of Hemovac and Staples
	13	Ann's Bandages Removed
	18-19	Writers' Conference in Calgary
	20	Removal of Catheter
	25-26	Discouraging Weekend
May	3	First Sense of Recovery

Prostate Cancer: My Story of Survival

ABOUT THE AUTHOR

Bryan Norford grew up in the UK, making architecture his first profession. With his wife Ann and young family, he immigrated to Canada in 1965 where he continued his architectural profession. Later he obtained a Master of Divinity degree at Regent College, Vancouver in 1982. He then pastored churches and taught in Bible colleges for several years in the lower mainland where he published a series of study guides on apologetics, ethics, and Bible surveys.

He is now retired and living in Lethbridge, Alberta where he and Ann authored their first book, *Happy Together, Daily Insights for Families from Scripture*, published in 2009. Bryan authored further books, *Guess Who's Coming to Reign! Jesus Talks about His return*, in 2010 and *Gone with the Spirit: Tracking the Holy Spirit through the Bible*, in 2011, and continues to write. Further materials are on his website at www.norfords-writings.com.

Ann and Bryan enjoy their writing activities, and spending time with their expanding family of grandchildren and great grandchildren.

Made in the USA
Charleston, SC
28 August 2012